CW00524128

HOMOEOPATHIC REMEDIES
FOR
EARS, NOSE and THROAT

HOMOEOPATHIC REMEDIES
FOR
EARS, NOSE and THROAT

by
Phyllis Speight

The C. W. Daniel Company Limited
Saffron Walden, Essex

Other books by Phyllis Speight

Arnica The Wonder Herb
Before Calling the Doctor
Comparison of the Chronic Miasms
Homoeopathy – A Practical Guide to
Natural Medicine
Overcoming Rheumatism & Arthritis
Pertinent Questions and Answers about
Homoeopathy
A Study Course in Homoeopathy
Homoeopathic Remedies for Children
Homoeopathy for Emergencies
A Travellers' Guide to Homoeopathy

First published in Great Britain by
The C. W. Daniel Company Limited
© Phyllis Speight 1990

ISBN 0 85207 217 1

Set by MS Typesetting, Castle Camps, Cambridge
and printed by Hillman Printers (Frome) Ltd,
Frome, Somerset

CONTENTS

PREFACE

I am delighted to learn that my books have introduced many people to homoeopathy and that they are helping their families, and especially their children, to become more healthy and therefore, happier people.

Many years of practice have given me the opportunity to observe what homoeopathy can achieve and I hope this book will enable readers to deal successfully with troubles that are in the acute stages and thus bring about healing speedily and avoid prolonged suffering.

This will probably be my last book (unless I have another urge) and I would like to say thank you to my husband for his help and support. Leslie is full of ideas and has always been my fiercest critic — 'If I cannot understand what you say, there isn't much hope for people with little or no knowledge of homoeopathy' he has said to me on many occasions! **And** he has typed all my manuscripts. I really am grateful!

I would also like to thank Ian Miller for promising to publish yet another book of mine — I feel it is so important to introduce homoeopathy and the correct way of applying it. So, thank you again Ian.

Phyllis Speight
Devon, 1990

1

INTRODUCTION

Homoeopathy is a complete system of medicine which has been in use since the 1880s.

It is based on the Law of Similars – Similia Similibus Curentur – let likes be cured by likes – in other words a remedy that will produce symptoms when taken by a healthy person will cure similar symptoms suffered by a sick person.

In order to ascertain the action of remedies they have been 'proved' on healthy men and women; in other words they took doses of a remedy under the supervision of a doctor until symptoms appeared. These were noted and collated and form the materia medicas from which we work today.

Homoeopaths treat patients by matching their symptoms to those produced by the remedy.

For instance, Nux vomica produced symptoms of a very irritable, fiery temperament; great excitement and impatience, anger and spitefulness. Great chilliness, even when hugging the fire and wearing layers of clothes; worse in the morning and in cold weather, also from over-eating and over-drinking. Better in warm, wet weather, in the evening, and after a nap. This, of course, is very brief but if a patient is unwell, cannot get warm and will bite your head off at the least thing, then Nux vomica would be the first remedy to come to mind.

The following pages should be studied carefully in order that the most similar remedy to the symptoms of the patient may be found.

With patience and care many troubles can be dealt with successfully but in a book of this size the number of remedies has to be limited. So if there is no real improvement within a reasonable time then the skills of an experienced homoeopath should be sought.

NOTES ABOUT
THE REMEDIES

Time is well spent in studying the homoeopathic remedies included in this book as they are some of the most commonly used for ear, nose and throat troubles.

In the pages on materia medica each remedy commences with 'characteristic' symptoms. These are very well defined symptoms which are found only in that particular remedy or they are symptoms which are more pronounced in that remedy than in any other.

They are not necessarily ear, nose or throat symptoms but may apply to the patient as a whole. When a remedy covering the physical symptoms has been found the remedy should be read through and if any characteristic symptoms apply this emphasizes that the prescription is correct.

At the end of each remedy there is a list of 'modalities' – anything that makes the patient or his symptoms better or worse. They are very important and should always be studied as an aid to remedy selection.

Following the materia medica is a small repertory which consists of lists of Characteristic symptoms under two headings – those of the mind and others which are 'general'.

Modalities follow and they come under four headings: –

Worse or aggravated by weather conditions.
Worse or aggravated by general conditions.
Better or ameliorated by weather conditions.
Better or ameliorated by general conditions.

Then there are lists of: –

Symptoms of the ear.
Symptoms of the nose.
Symptoms of the throat.

These lists should enable the prescriber to look up symptoms quickly and match them to the remedy, but before actually prescribing **always read the remedy in the materia medica to confirm your choice**.

HOW TO FIND THE CORRECT REMEDY

There are many homoeopathic remedies covering symptoms of ear-ache, noises in the ear,
nose stopped up or running; sneezing; sore
throat; difficulty in swallowing; swelling of
tonsils and so on.

None of the above symptoms would lead us to
a remedy as they are too 'common' and have
nothing to identify them. More information can
be obtained by asking the patient questions
according to the following guide lines. The
answers should be written down.

1. LOCATION

Where exactly is the trouble? This should be
described in the patient's own words − e.g.

Which ear − internal, external etc.

The right or left nostril or both, or at the back
of the nose etc.

Position of pain or swelling in throat.

2. SENSATION

A description of the pain or discomfort, e.g.,
throbbing, soreness, blocked up sensation, pain
on swallowing etc.

Describe or ask the patient to describe the
sensation in his own words. Never try to
answer on behalf of anybody else.

When a baby is involved observation plays the biggest part.

MODALITY

This is anything that makes the symptoms better or worse.
e.g., throbbing pain in left ear better for warmth; sticking pain in throat better for swallowing.

With this information it should be possible to match the 'picture' with a remedy which has similar symptoms.

The following examples may prove helpful: –
1. A child suddenly complains of earache after being out in a very cold wind, which is worse when lying on it.

Aconite comes to mind – look it up and you will see why.
2. An adult develops a bad cold with copious yellow mucus and a feeling of pressure at the root of the nose. These symptoms are worse in a warm, stuffy room and better in fresh air for which she craves.

Look at Pulsatilla and you will see why this will help her.
3. A young man complained of a very sore throat with burning which is worse on the right side. He wants to swallow constantly and when he does he feels a stitching sensation up into the ear. He is worse at night and in a warm bed.

Mercurius would help the patient, look it up for details.

POTENCY AND DOSE
OF HOMOEOPATHIC
REMEDIES

Homoeopathic remedies are prepared in a special way by homoeopathic pharmacists and should always be purchased from a reliable firm.

They are sensitive and should be kept in a drawer or cupboard away from sunlight and strong smelling perfumes or soaps, etc.

Pills or tablets should be handled as little as possible – usually they can be shaken into the cap of the container and popped into the mouth.

One pill or tablet is sufficient and is one dose. Put it under the tongue where it will dissolve quickly; do **not** wash it down with water and it should not be taken immediately after cleaning the teeth with a flavoured toothpaste.

In acute troubles remedies may be given frequently in the 6th or 12th potency – half-hourly if necessary for up to three doses and then less frequently, two or three hourly until symptoms improve; but the frequency of the dose depends on the severity of the condition. This dosage is only a guide and discretion should be used according to the needs of the patient. Potencies higher than the 12th should not be used by those with no experience of homoeopathy.

The golden rule in every case is that as soon as the patient begins to improve doses must be given less frequently and stopped altogether when symptoms disappear. This is a strict rule which must be adhered to.

If after a few hours there is no improvement then a re-assessment must be made and another search for a different remedy. This high-lights the importance of study in order to find the correct remedy because it is not a good idea to change the remedy several times hoping that in the end the right one will be found. Remember, a sick person needs to be cured in the shortest possible time.

If there is no sign of improvement or the condition gets worse, then a doctor should be consulted without delay.

LIST OF REMEDIES

Aconitum Napellus	Monkshood
Ammonium Carbonicum	Sal Volatile
Argentum Nitricum	Silver
Arsenicum Album	White Arsenic
Belladonna	Deadly Nightshade
Calcarea Carbonica	Secretion of the Oyster shell
Causticum	Potassium Hydrate
Gelsemium	Yellow Jasmine
Graphites	Black Lead
Kali Bichromicum	Bichromate of Potash
Kali Carbonicum	Carbonate of Potassium Potash
Lachesis	The Surukuku Snake
Lycopodium	Club Moss
Mercurius Solubis	Mercury
Natrum Muriaticum	Sodium Chloride – Common Salt
Nitric Acid	
Nux Vomica	Poison Nut
Petroleum	Rock Oil
Phosphorus	Made from Bone-Ash
Phytolacca Decandra	Pokeroot

Pulsatilla	Pasque flower – Anemone
Rhus Toxicodendron	Poison Nut
Sanguinaria	Blood-root
Sepia	Liquid from the Ink Sac of Cuttlefish
Silica	Silicon Dioxide
Sulphur	Brimstone

REMEDIES AND
THEIR ABBREVIATIONS

Aconitum Napellus	*Acon.*
Ammonium Carbonicum	*Amm.c.*
Argentum Nitricum	*Arg.n.*
Arsenicum album	*Ars.a.*
Belladonna	*Bell.*
Calcarea Carbonica	*Calc.c.*
Causticum	*Caust.*
Gelsemium	*Gels.*
Graphites	*Graph.*
Kali Bichromicum	*Kali b.*
Kali Carbonicum	*Kali c.*
Lachesis	*Lach.*
Lycopodium	*Lyc.*
Mercurius Solubilis	*Merc.s.*
Natrum Muriaticum	*Nat.m.*
Nitric Acid	*Nit.a.*
Nux Vomica	*Nux v.*
Petroleum	*Petr.*
Phosphorus	*Phos.*
Phytolacca Decandra	*Phyt.*
Pulsatilla	*Puls.*
Rhus Toxicodendron	*Rhus t.*
Sanguinaria	*Sang.*
Sepia	*Sep.*

| Silica | *Sil.* |
| Sulphur | *Sulph.* |

ACONITE

Characteristics

Fear, anxiety, physical and mental restlessness.
Fright – Aconite has a calming effect.
The sudden beginning of an acute illness with fever and anxiety, restlessness and fear.
Fearful of the future, of death, there are so many fears.
Can vomit with fear.
There is much tension.

EARS: Very sensitive to noise.
Earache, stitching and tearing pains.
External ear hot, red, painful and swollen.
Feels as though a drop of water is in the ear.
Buzzing, ringing, humming and roaring noises.

NOSE: Should be given at the very beginning of a cold, at the very first sensation of burning, tingling or sneezing.
Frequent sneezing; dropping of clear, hot water from nostrils.
Mucous membranes dry; nose stopped up.
Dry or with scanty, watery mucus.
Pain at root of nose.
Smell acutely sensitive.

THROAT: Red, dry, hot, constricted.
Burning, smarting, dryness and tingling in throat which is **very** red.
Swallowing hurts; sometimes cannot swallow.
Uvula feels long.

14

Tonsils swollen and dry.
Larynx sensitive.
Hoarseness.
There may be a high fever with great thirst for cold water.

MODALITIES:
Worse: Warm room; around midnight; tobacco smoke; music; cold, dry winds.
Better: Open air.
Note: Complaints caused by exposure to dry, cold winds.

AMMONIUM CARBONICUM

Characteristics
Weak, anaemic, flabby.
Weakness with no reaction.
Faintness.
Nosebleed whilst washing the face.

EARS: Hardness of hearing.
Itching.
Buzzing noise.

NOSE: Stoppage at night with long continued coryza.
Cannot breathe through nose.
Snuffles of children.
Bloody mucus.
Itching in nose.
Epitaxis whilst washing the face.

THROAT: Sore, raw feeling.
Enlarged tonsils and glands of neck.
Tendency to ulceration of tonsils.
Burning pains.
Hoarseness.

MODALITIES:
Worse: Evening, cold wet weather; wet applications; from 3 a.m. to 4 a.m.

Better: Lying on painful side and on stomach; dry weather.

ARGENTUM NITRICUM

Characteristics
Impulsive, wants to do things in a hurry. Must walk fast.
Time passes slowly.
Nervous and apprehensive, sometimes has an attack of diarrhoea, especially before going to theatre or church.
Great desire for sugar.

EARS: Buzzing in ears with vertigo.
Ringing noise with deafness.
Tearing and stitching pains in ears.
Hearing lost.

NOSE: Nose running, feels chilly with headache.
Violent itching.
Loss of smell.

THROAT: Much thick tenacious mucus causing hawking.
Rawness, soreness and scraping causing hawking and cough.
Sensation of splinter, worse swallowing and better cold drinks.
Strangulated feeling.
Catarrh of smokers.
Chronic hoarseness.

MODALITIES:
Worse: Warmth in any form; at night; from sweets; cold food; after eating; at menstrual period; from emotion; left side.
Better: From eructations; pressure; cold air; patient craves fresh air.

ARSENICUM ALBUM

Characteristics

Great anguish and restlessness.

Fear, fright and worry.

Prostration yet marked restlessness from anxiety making patient change places constantly.

Great exhaustion after slightest exertion.

Fastidious, hates disorder.

Burning pains better by heat but patient always wants the head kept cool.

Burning discharges.

Great thirst for small quantities at frequent intervals.

EARS: Thin, excoriating, offensive otorrhoea.

Roaring, ringing and singing noises.

Burning, stitching and tearing pains.

Hearing impaired; human voice difficult to hear.

NOSE: Thin, watery, excoriating discharge which excoriates upper lip.

Sneezing from intense tickle inside nose.

Nose stopped up, not relieved by sneezing.

Sneezing from every change in weather.

Burning sensation.

Colds begin in nose and go down to chest.

Nose bleed after anger or vomiting.

Acne of nose.

THROAT: Swollen, burning, difficulty in swallowing.

MODALITIES:

Worse: Cold air; wet weather; cold drinks; cold applications; night; after midnight, 1 a.m. to 3 a.m.

Better: Warmth (except head); loves and craves heat.

BELLADONNA

Characteristics

This remedy stands for HEAT, REDNESS, THROBBING and BURNING.

Attacks are violent and onset sudden.

Many acute local inflammations; fevers with hot, burning, dry skin, so hot that heat can be felt by the hand before it touches the skin.

Very red, flushed face; dilated pupils of the eyes.

Sudden rise in temperature.

Fears imaginary things, wants to escape; run away.

Starts in fright when approached.

Restless sleep from excited mental states which can go on to delirium.

There is often an acuteness of all senses.

Can get very angry.

EARS: Tearing, boring, pressing pains in middle and external ear.

Pains can cause delirium.

Child cries out in sleep; pain throbbing and beating deep in ear.

Buzzing, humming, ringing, roaring noises.

Acute condition of eustachian tube.

Hearing impaired; sometimes lost.

Otitis media.

NOSE: Red, swollen, sore and hot.

Bleeding of nose with red face.

Mucus mixed with blood.

Not much discharge.

Sudden onset of colds.

THROAT: Dry as if glazed; inflamed and bright red; worse right side and going to left; feels constricted; raw and sore.

Tonsils enlarged; tonsillitis.

Swallowing difficult, worse liquids.

Continual inclination to swallow.

18

Spasm on trying to swallow so that food and liquids come back through the nose.
Dryness of fauces.

MODALITIES:
Worse: After 3 p.m. or after midnight; from uncovering, or draft of air and lying down; touch; jar; noise; draught.
Better: Being semi-erect (with head high) and being covered.

CALCAREA CARBONICA

Characteristics
Fat, flabby, fair, faint.
Apprehensive and has every kind of fear.
Hand is soft, cool and boneless; gives you the shivers to shake hands with Calcarea.
Everything smells sour, stool, sweat, urine, and taste is sour.
Profuse cold, sour sweat, especially on head.
Sweats even in cold room.
Enlargement of glands.
Craves eggs and indigestible things like chalk, earth, raw potatoes.
Feels better when constipated.
Feet feel as if wearing cold, damp stockings.
Great sensitivity to cold and cold, damp weather, dreads open air; at the same time cannot bear the sun.
Breathlessness; walking slowly up a slight hill can bring on sweating and breathlessness.

EARS: Throbbing, cracking, stitching pains.
Pulsating and feeling as if something was coming out of ear.
Buzzing, hissing, ringing, roaring and surging noises.
Hardness of hearing; deafness from working in water.
Muco-purulent otorrhoea and enlarged glands.

Eruption on and behind ears.
Sensitive to cold about ears and neck.

NOSE: Takes cold at every change of weather, with much sneezing. Swelling of nose and upper lip.
Sneezes often without a cold.
Nostrils dry and sore, ulcerated.
Lingering catarrh with thick, fetid, yellow discharge. Great crusts from nose.
Nose gets stuffed up during the night.
Nose bleed in children inclined to be fat.
Polypi with loss of smell; swelling at root of nose.

THROAT: Swelling of tonsils and sub-maxillary glands. Uvula swollen.
Hawks up mucus.
Small ulcers spreading to palate.
Goitre.

MODALITIES:
Worse: On waking; morning; after midnight; bathing; working in water; full moon; mental and physical exertion; stooping; pressure of clothes; open air; cold air; cold wet weather; letting limbs hang down.
Better: After breakfast; drawing up limbs; loosening garments; in the dark; lying on back; from rubbing; dry, warm weather.

CAUSTICUM

Characteristics
Intensely sympathetic.
Depression, apprehension, timidity, irritability.
Aches and pains with soreness, rawness and burning.
Paralysis of single parts, e.g. face, throat, vocal chords, limbs, from exposure to cold, dry winds.
Skin dirty white, sallow.

EARS: Many noises – ringing, roaring, pulsating with deafness.
Also buzzing, humming, reverberating.
Hearing impaired or even lost.
Words and steps re-echo in ears.
Pains inside ears which can be burning, pressing, stitching, tearing, pulsating.
Stopped-up feeling.
Accumulation of wax which can be offensive.
Chronic middle ear catarrh.

NOSE: Coryza with hoarseness.
Dry coryza with stoppage of nose.
Fluent coryza with pain in chest and limbs.
Violent bleeding of nose.
Itching tip of nose.
Pimples and warts on nose.

THROAT: Pains burning with rawness and soreness.
Pain worse stooping.
Rawness and tickling with dry cough.
Dryness, constantly obliged to swallow.
Mucus collects which cannot be raised.
Hoarseness, larynx sore.

MODALITIES:
Worse: Dry, cold winds; in fine clear weather; cold air.
Better: Damp, wet weather; warmth.

GELSEMIUM

Characteristics
Affects more the nerves of motion, causing muscular prostration and varying degrees of motor paralysis.
Dizziness, drowsiness, dullness, trembling.
Tiredness, limbs feel tired; eyelids feel heavy.
Fearful; terrors of anticipation.
Apathy regarding illness.

EARS: Swallowing causes pain in ear.

NOSE: Coryza some days after exposure with severe sneezing in early morning and a profuse flow of scalding watery discharge.
Nostrils sore. There is often a blockage at root of nose.
Catarrhs of warm, moist, relaxing weather.

THROAT: Sore — tonsils red, difficulty in swallowing because of weak throat muscles.
Symptoms develop gradually with muscular weakness.
Feels rough and burning.
Feeling of lump in throat that cannot be swallowed.
Tonsillitis.
Itching and tickling in soft palate and naso-pharynx.
Aphonia, either nervous or catarrhal in origin.

MODALITIES:
Worse: Damp weather; emotion; excitement; bad news: 10 a.m.
Better: Bending forward; open air; continued motion; headache is relieved by profuse urination.

GRAPHITES

Characteristics
Fat — Chilly — Costive.
Has an affinity with women who are overweight, chilly and constipated.
Obesity.
Music causes patient to cry.
Intolerance of light, especially sunlight.
Very rough skin with cracks.
Eruptions oozing sticky, honey-like substance.
Always cold but craves fresh air, must be well wrapped up.

On the other hand she suffers when the weather is very hot.

EARS: Dryness of inner ear.
Hardness of hearing; hears better in noise.
Hissing noise.
Fissures in and behind ears.
Moisture and eruptions behind ears.

NOSE: Sore on blowing. Painful internally.
Dryness, scabs and fissures in nostrils.
Stopped up with badly smelling mucus.
Smell abnormally acute.

THROAT: Hoarseness, especially on beginning to sing and while voice is breaking.
Inability to control the vocal chords.

MODALITIES:
Worse: Warmth at night.
Better: In the dark; wrapping up.

KALI BICHROMICUM

Characteristics
Discharge of tough, stringy, adherent mucus or jelly-like mucus.
Pain comes in small spots.

EARS: Swollen with tearing pain.
Chronic suppuration of ear.
Thick, yellow, fetid, stringy, tenacious discharge, often more mucus than pus.
Sharp stitches in ear.
Ear-drum perforated.

NOSE: Profuse watery nasal discharge.
Violent sneezing.
Coryza with obstruction in nose.
Snuffles of children, especially, fat, chubby babies.

23

Inflammation extends to frontal sinuses with distress and pressing pains at root of nose, and over eyes.

Discharge of clinkers, plugs.

Chronic inflammation of frontal sinuses.

Septum ulcerated, round ulcer, fetid smell.

Discharge thick, ropy (can be drawn out in strings),greenish-yellow; or tough and jelly-like. Offensive.

Catarrh dropping from posterior nares.

Much hawking, inability to breathe through nose.

Loss of smell.

THROAT: Dry and rough.

Fauces red and inflamed.

Hawking of thick gelatinous mucus, worse morning.

Deep ulcers of fauces.

Parotid glands swollen.

Pseudo membranous deposits on tonsils and soft palate.

Discharge from mouth to throat tough and stringy.

Has cleared up cases of diphtheria when symptoms agreed.

Voice hoarse.

MODALITIES:
Worse: Morning; hot weather; undressing.
Better: from heat.

KALI CARBONICUM

Characteristics
Very irritable.

Anxiety felt in the stomach.

Fearful. Hates to be touched; and being alone.

Hypersensitive to pain, noise and touch.

All pains are sharp, cutting.

Stitches may be felt in any part of the body.

Intolerance of cold weather.

EARS: Stitches in ears; itching; cracking, ringing and roaring noises.
A curious sensation as if 'cold air is blowing into ear' may be noticed.

NOSE: Stuffs up in a warm room.
Discharge is thick, fluent, yellow, and is often post-nasal.
Nostrils are ulcerated, sore and scurfy.
Nose can be swollen, hard and red from tip to root.

THROAT: Always taking cold which settles in the throat.
Dry, parched and rough.
Pains stinging when swallowing and often a sticking pain as from a fishbone.
Swallowing is difficult.
Accumulation of mucus in the morning.

MODALITIES:
Worse: From soup and coffee; at 3 a.m.; lying on left and painful side.
Better: In warm, moist weather; moving about.

LACHESIS

Characteristics
Insanely jealous and suspicious. Anxious.
Loquacity.
Worse from sleep. Sleeps into an aggravation (no matter what the symptoms).
Worse left side. Sometimes moving to the right.
Intolerance of anything tight, especially round neck or waist.

EARS: Tearing pain from cheekbone into ear, also with sore throat.
Ear wax hard and dry.

NOSE: Bleeding – nostrils sensitive.
Coryza preceded by headaches.
Hay-asthma – paroxysms of sneezing.

THROAT: Sore, worse left side and swallowing liquids.
Chronic sore throat with much hawking of mucus which sticks and cannot be forced up or down. Very painful, worse slightest pressure; worse swallowing saliva or liquids.
Hawking of mucus with rawness of throat, worse after a nap during the day.
Dry throat in night and on waking.
Pain in throat in connection with ears.
Throat swollen with sensation as if full of crumbs.
Throat and larynx painful when bending head back.
Sore and ulcerated.
Sensitive with pain on left side.
Empty swallowing or swallowing of saliva or liquids aggravates more than the swallowing of solids.
Very sensitive to external pressure.
Septic parotiditis.
Diphtheric membrane dusky, blackish; pain worse hot drinks.
Quinsy.
Collar and neck band must be very loose.

MODALITIES:
Worse: After sleep; left side; in the spring; pressure or constriction; hot drinks.
Better: Warm applications; the appearance of any discharge.

LYCOPODIUM

Characteristics
Intellectually keen but physically weak.
Upper part of body thin, lower part dropsical.

Very apprehensive – anticipation – before delivering address, lecture; etc., but fine as soon as she gets going.

Likes to be alone but somebody in the next room or other part of the house.

Weeps when thanked.

Good appetite but a few mouthfuls fills up and she feels bloated.

Excessive accumulation of wind in lower abdomen.

Fullness – flatulence – distension.

Symptoms begin on right side and often move to the left.

Craves sweets.

EARS: Thick, yellow, offensive discharge.

Tearing pain inside ears.

Stopped up sensation.

Hearing impaired, sometimes lost.

Otorrhoea and deafness with or without tinnitus.

Humming and roaring with deafness.

NOSE: Fluent coryza.

Nose stopped up with catarrh, cannot breathe.

Violent catarrh with swelling of nose.

Ulcerated nostrils – crusts and elastic plugs.

Child starts from sleep rubbing nose.

Fan-like motion of alae nasi.

Sense of smell very acute.

THROAT: Dryness without thirst.

Inflammation of throat with stitches on swallowing, better warm drinks.

Feels too tight on swallowing.

Swelling and suppuration of tonsils beginning on right side.

Diphtheria, deposits spread from right to left, worse cold drinks.

Ulceration of vocal bands.

Feeling as if a ball rose from below up into throat.

MODALITIES:

Worse: 4 to 8 p.m. (no other remedy has this as such an outstanding symptom); cold food and drink; oysters; warm room.

Better: Warm food and drink (and much prefers it); open air; Movement.

MERCURIUS SOLUBILIS

Characteristics

Hasty – hurried – restless – anxious – impulsive.

Trembling.

Weakness.

Sweats without relief.

Profuse perspiration which does not relieve.

Salivation with intense thirst.

Mouth offensive – tongue large, flabby, shows imprint of teeth.

EARS: Inflamed internally and externally with sticking pain; feels stopped up.

Bloody and offensive discharge from right ear.

Pains inside ear can be pulsating, tearing, burning, pressing.

Thick yellow discharge.

Earache worse warmth of bed at night.

Boils in external canal.

Hearing impaired with tearing pain.

NOSE: Much violent sneezing, fluent corrosive greenish-yellow, offensive discharge. Nose drips. Sore, raw, smarting sensation.

Nostrils raw, ulcerated; nasal bones swollen.

Acrid, yellow-green, fetid, pus-like discharge.

Copious discharge of corroding mucus.

Coryza, acrid discharge but too thick to run down lips, worse in a warm room.

Pain and swelling of nasal bones and caries with greenish, fetid ulceration.

Catarrhal inflammation of frontal sinuses.

Nose red, swollen, shining.
Nose bleed.

THROAT: Sore throat accompanies every cold.
Throat feels dry and swallowing is painful, but must keep swallowing because of free flow of saliva.
When swallowing, shooting pain in tonsils.
Stitches into ear on swallowing.
Suppuration of tonsils with sharp, sticking pain in fauces when swallowing.
Putrid sore throat, worse right side.
Bluish-red swelling.
Sore, raw, smarting, burning pains.
Burning as from hot vapour.
Ulcers and inflammation appearing at every change in weather.
Quinsy with difficult swallowing after pus has formed.
Complete loss of voice.

MODALITIES:
Worse: Night; warmth of bed; while sweating; lying on right side.

NATRUM MURIATICUM

Characteristics
Ill effects of grief, fright, anger.
Consolation aggravates; wants to be alone to cry.
Depressed; moody.
Very irritable.
Great weakness and weariness.
All mucous membranes dry.
Craves salt.
Very thirsty.

EARS: Noises – roaring, ringing, cracking in ears when chewing.

NOSE: Violent, fluent coryza lasting 1-3 days, then changing into stoppage of nose making breathing difficult.

Discharge thin, watery like raw white of egg.

Violent sneezing coryza.

Internal soreness of nose.

Dryness.

Loss of smell and taste.

Good for emotional type of cold with much watery sneezing.

Infallible for stopping a cold commencing with sneezing (Boericke).

Chronic nasal catarrh.

THROAT: Chronic naso-pharyngeal catarrh worse in the morning with much hawking of mucus.

Hoarseness with persistent tickle causing a cough.

The throat may feel plugged and there is a sensation of lump on swallowing food.

MODALITIES:
Worse: Noise; music; 10 a.m. to 11 a.m.; consolation; sea-shore (can be better sea-shore); heat of sun or heat in general.
Better: Open air; cold bathing; sweating.

NITRIC ACID

Characteristics
Irritability.
Pains as from splinters.
Sticking pains.

EARS: Difficult hearing, worse riding in carriage or train.
Very sensitive to noise.
Cracking in ears when chewing.

NOSE: Ozoena, green casts from nose every morning.

Paroxysms of sneezing.

Coryza with sore, bleeding nostrils.

Chronic catarrh with yellow, offensive, corrosive discharge, causing swelling of upper lip, acrid and watery at night.

Watery vesicles around lips and nose.

Stitches as of splinter in nose.

Ulceration of nostrils; inner nose scurfy with frequent bleeding.

Nosebleed with chest infections.

Tip of nose red.

THROAT: Dry. Hawks mucus constantly.

Swallowing very difficult; cannot swallow even a teaspoonful of fluid as it causes violent pain extending to ear.

A feeling of splinters in throat on swallowing.

Stinging pains in swollen throat.

Tonsils swollen, red and uneven with small ulcers.

White patches on throat.

MODALITIES:

Worse: Cold climate and also in hot weather.

NUX VOMICA

Characteristics

Very anxious, irritable, fiery temperament, impatient.

Can get excited, angry, spiteful and malicious.

Very particular and careful people.

Easily offended; anxious; depressed.

Sullen; fault-finding.

Over-sensitive to slightest noise; strong odours; bright light; music. Feels everything too strongly.

Quick in movement.

Very chilly and when unwell in spite of layers of clothing and hugging the fire, still feels cold.

EARS: Itching in ear through eustachian tube.

Auditory canal dry and sensitive.
Diminishes sensation of auditory nerves; loud sounds are painful and make patient angry.

NOSE: Stuffed up, especially at night.
Stuffy colds, snuffles after exposure to dry, cold atmosphere, worse in warm room.
Coryza fluent in day-time, stuffed up at night and out of doors or alternates between nostrils.
Streams in warm room during day but rather better out of doors.
Sneezing after meals.
Coryza with scraping in throat and sneezing.
Dry weather type of cold; patient is full of flatulence and resentment.
Acrid discharge but with stuffed up feeling.

THROAT: Rough, scraped feeling from catarrh.
Throat sore with raw feeling that promotes a cough.
Sensation of roughness, tightness and tension.
Pharynx constricted.
Uvula swollen.
Stitches in ear.

MODALITIES:
Worse: Cold; dry winds; east winds; morning; over-eating; over-drinking.
Better: Warm, wet weather; evening; after a nap.

PETROLEUM

Characteristics
Skin eruptions worse in winter.

EARS: Noise unbearable, especially from several people talking simultaneously.
Dry catarrh with deafness and noises.

Chronic eustachian catarrh.
Eustachian tubes affected causing whizzing, roaring and cracking noises with hardness of hearing.
Diminished hearing.
Eczema in and behind ears with intense itching, redness and soreness.
Parts sore to touch.

NOSE: Nostrils ulcerated, cracked, burning; tip of nose itching.
Nose bleeds.
Ozoena with scabs and muco-purulent discharge.
Pustules in nose.

MODALITIES:
Worse: In winter (skin eruptions).
Better: In summer (skin eruptions).

PHOSPHORUS

Characteristics
Extremely sensitive, especially to external impressions.
Fearful of thunderstorms; being alone; of the dark; disease; death; that something awful will happen.
Very affectionate; they need it and give it, yet there can be an indifference.
Desire to be rubbed.
Much weakness and trembling.
Burning pains.
Haemorrhages bright and freely flowing.
Thirst for cold drinks which are vomited as soon as they become warm in the stomach.

EARS: Hearing difficult, especially the human voice.
Re-echoing sounds.

NOSE: Fan-like motion of nostrils.

Epitaxis instead of periods.

Oversensitive to smell.

The stopping and starting type of cold; frequent alternations of fluent and stopped coryza.

Discharge from one nostril and stoppage of the other.

Chronic catarrh with small haemorrhages – handkerchief always bloody.

Polypi – bleeding easily.

Inflammation of the membrane covering the nasal bones.

THROAT: Pain from sneezing.

MODALITIES:

Worse: Physical or mental exertion; twilight; warm food or drink; from getting wet in hot weather; change of weather; evening; lying on painful side.

Better: Heat (everywhere except stomach and head).

Dr. Margaret Tyler says: 'Phosphorus complaints are worse from cold and cold weather, better from heat and warm applications, except for the complaints of head and stomach, which are ameliorated from cold'.

PHYTOLACCA

Characteristics

Irresistible inclinations to bite teeth or gums together.

EARS: Shooting pains, especially on right side, worse by swallowing.

NOSE: Coryza; with pain at root of nose.

One nostril becomes alternately blocked or discharges acrid, excoriating mucus. Or nose may be totally blocked; this is not eased by blowing.

THROAT: Dark red or bluish red.

Sensation of a lump in throat; as if a red hot iron was stuck in throat.

Sore, congested, bright red.

Tonsils red, swollen with white spots, worse right side.

Shooting pains into ears, often on swallowing.

Cannot swallow anything hot.

Cannot swallow, even water.

Dryness, roughness, burning and smarting of fauces.

Pseudo membranous exudation, grayish-white; thick tenacious, yellowish mucus difficult to dislodge.

Ulcerated sore throat. Diphtheria.

Throat feels very hot; pain at root of tongue extending to ear.

Uvula enlarged.

Quinsy; tonsils and fauces swollen with burning pain.

Mumps.

Voice gives out from over-work and there is much burning in throat as of a hot substance there.

MODALITIES:
Worse: On motion but must move, he aches and is so sore.

PULSATILLA

Characteristics
The temperament is mild and gentle but anger can appear, and irritability.
Tears come very easily.
Conscientious, hates to be hussled.
Loves sympathy and fuss.

Changeable in everything; in disposition (like an April shower and sunshine); pains wander from joint to joint; no two stools are alike, etc.

Pulsatilla feels the heat; they must have air; it makes them feel much better.

Cannot eat fat, rich food, it makes them feel sick.

Thirstless, even with a fever.

EARS: Sensation as if something was being forced outward.

Hearing difficulties as if ear was stuffed up.

Diminished acuteness of hearing.

Otorrhoea.

Thick, bland discharge; offensive odour.

Catarrhal otitis.

Earache worse at night.

External ear swollen and red.

NOSE: Coryza, stoppage of right nostril, pressing pain at root of nose.

Stuffing up of nose at night and copious flow in the morning. Fluent in open air, stopped up indoors.

Thick, yellow, bland mucus out of doors, abundant in morning.

Old catarrh with loss of smell.

Nasal bones sore.

Large green fetid scales.

Alae nasi ulcerated externally and exude watery fluid.

THROAT: Painful as if raw; sore throat, scratchy, dry.

MODALITIES:
Worse: Warm room; warm applications. Cannot bear heat in any form.
Better: Cool open air; walking slowly in open air but pains of Pulsatilla are accompanied by chilliness.

RHUS TOXICODENDRON

Characteristics

Great restlessness; cannot lie or sit long in one position. Changes often for temporary relief.
Stiffness on beginning to move.
Triangular red-tip of tongue.

EARS: Pain with sensation as if something were in them, lobules swollen.
Discharge of bloody pus.

NOSE: Sneezing, coryza from getting wet.
Nose stopped up with every cold.
Mucus runs from nose in morning, after rising.
Frequent violent, spasmodic sneezing.
Tip of nose red, sore, ulcerated.
Swelling of nose.
Nose bleed on stooping.

THROAT: Dryness with great thirst.
Sore with swollen glands.
Very swollen externally, maxilliary and parotid glands greatly enlarged.
Redness and oedema of throat.
Sticking pain on swallowing.
Parotitis left side.

MODALITIES:

Worse: Quietly sitting or lying and on beginning to move: lifting or straining; getting wet when sweating; wet, cold weather.
Better: By continued motion until tiredness sets in; warmth; dry air and weather.

SANGUINARIA

Characteristics

Pain in occiput, spreads over the head and settles over right eye.
Pain in right arm and shoulder.
Loose cough with badly smelling sputa.

EARS: Burning in ears with cough.
Earache with headache.
Humming and roaring in ears.
Aurul polypi.

NOSE: Oezena with profuse, offensive, yellowish discharges.
Hay fever.
Coryza followed by diarrhoea.
Chronic rhinitis, membrane dry and congested.
Nasal polypi.

THROAT: Swollen, worse right side.
Dry and constricted.
Ulceration of mouth and fauces with dry, burning sensation.
Tonsillitis.

MODALITIES:
Worse: Right side (symptoms).

SEPIA

Characteristics
Great indifference to family (to husband and often children) and friends.
Averse to work; loses interest in what she ordinarily loves.
Irritable.
Easily offended.
Anxious and fearful.
Dreads to be alone.
Nervous, jumpy, hysterical.
Weeps when telling symptoms.
Depressed. Hates sympathy and weeps if it is offered.
Wants to get away to be quiet.
Weakness; weariness.
Pains travel upwards.
A 'ball' sensation in inner parts.
Faint when kneeling.

Feels the cold, must have air.
Gnawing hunger.
Craves vinegar and sour things; aversion to meat, fat, often bread and milk.
Yellow saddle across upper cheeks and nose.

EARS: Pain as if sub-cutaneous ulceration.
Swelling and eruption of external ear.
Herpes behind ears on nape of neck.

NOSE: Thick, greenish discharge; thick plugs and crusts, with offensive smell.
Catarrh with greenish crusts from anterior nose and pain at root of nose.
Chronic nasal catarrh, especially post-nasal; dropping of heavy, lumpy discharge which must be hawked through the mouth.
Dry coryza; nostrils sore, swollen, ulcerated, scabby, discharging large green plugs.

MODALITIES:
Worse: Damp; left side; after sweating; cold; cold air; east winds; sultry, moist weather.
Better: Exercise; pressure; warmth of bed; hot applications.

SILICA

Characteristics
Want of grit — moral and physical.
Yielding, faint-hearted, anxious.
Very sensitive to all impressions.
Easily irritated over trifles; touchy and self-willed.
Fixed ideas.
Intolerance of alcohol.
Suppurative processes.
Under nourished from imperfect assimilation.

EARS: Fetid discharge.
Decay of mastoid.
Loud pistol-like reports.

Roaring in ears.
Sensitive to noise; loud sounds.

NOSE: Sneezing in morning.
Obstructed and loss of smell.
Dry, hard crusts form, bleeding when loosened.
Nasal bones sensitive and sore.
Perforation of septum.
Itching at point of nose.

THROAT: Colds settle in throat.
Pricking as if pin in tonsil.
Stinging pain when swallowing.
Parotid glands swollen.
Hard, cold swelling of cervical glands.
Periodical quinsy.

MODALITIES: Feels the cold.
Worse: Morning; uncovering; damp.
Better: Warmth; wrapping up head; in the summer; in wet or humid weather.

SULPHUR

Characteristics
This remedy is known as the ragged philosopher.
Selfish, lazy and untidy people who often fling themselves into a chair with one leg draped over the arm. They are philosophical, wanting to know the 'Why's and wherefore's'.
Skin burning with itching; worse from warmth of bed.
Red orifices; eyes, nose, ears, lips and anus.
Sinking feeling mid-morning.
Worse standing.
Discharges offensive, acrid and excoriating, making parts over which they flow red and burning.
Dislike of water; of washing.

Cat-nap sleep.

EARS: Bad effects from suppression of an otorrhoea.

Lancinating, stinging, tearing in ear extending to head and throat, worse by being disturbed, musical sounds and all voices.

Chronic otitis from a boil in meatus with purulent discharge, in children.

Deafness preceded by exceedingly sensitive hearing.

Catarrhal deafness.

Deafness worse after eating or blowing nose.

NOSE: Constant sneezing; fluent like water trickling from nose.

Discharge acrid and burning.

Chronic dry catarrh. Dry scabs readily bleeding.

Nose stopped up indoors.

Swelling and inflammation in nose.

Smell as of old catarrh.

Adenoids and polypi.

THROAT: Pressure as from a lump, feeling like a splinter or a hair in throat.

Burning, redness, dryness.

Dryness of throat exciting cough at night.

Stitches on swallowing; painful contraction.

Constant desire to swallow saliva.

Swelling of palate and tonsils; elongation of palate.

Ball seems to rise and close the pharynx.

MODALITIES:
Worse: Warmth of bed; morning.
Better: Dry, warm weather.

CHARACTERISTICS –
MIND

Affectionate – *Phos.*
Alone, likes to be, but somebody in the house
  – *Lyc.*
Anger – *Nat.m; Nux v.; Puls.*
Anguish – *Ars.a.*
Anticipation – *Gels; Lyc.*
Anxiety – *Acon.; Ars.a.; Kali c.; Lach.;*
  Merc.s.; Nux v.; Sep.
Apathy – *Gels.*
Apprehensive – *Arg.n.; Calc.c.; Caust.; Lyc.*
Averse to work – *Sep.*

Careful – *Nux v.*
Conscientious – *Puls.*
Consolation aggravates – *Nat.m.*

Depression – *Caust.; Nat.m.; nux v.; Sep.*
Dullness – *Gels.*

Excited – *Nux v.*
Excited mental state causing restless sleep –
  Bell.

Faint – *Calc.c.*
Faint when kneeling – *Sep.*
Fastidious – *Ars.a.*
Fault-finding – *Nux v.*
Fearful – *Acon.; Ars.a.; Bell.; Calc.c.; Gels.;*
  Kali c.; Phos.; Sep.
Fiery – *Nux v.*

Fixed ideas – *Sil.*
Fright – *Acon.; Ars.a.; Bell.; Nat.m.*

Gentle – *Puls.*
Grief – *Nat.m.*
Grit, lacks moral – *Sil.*

Hurried – *Arg.n.; Merc.s.; Nux v.*
Hypersensitive – *Kali c.; Nux v.; Phos.*
Hysterical – *Sep.*

Impatient – *Nux v.*
Impulsive – *Arg.n.; Merc.s.*
Indifferent – *Sep.*
Irritable – *Caust.; Kali c.; Nat.m.; Nit.a.; Nux v.; Puls.; Sep.; Sil.*
Irritated over trifles – *Sil.*

Jealous – *Lach.*
Jumpy – *Sep.*

Lazy – *Sulph.*

Malicious – *Nux v.*
Moods changing – *Nat.m.; Puls.*

Nervous – *Arg.n.; Sep.*

Offended, easily – *Nux v.; Sep.*

Particular – *Nux v.*

Restlessness – *Acon.; Ars.a.; Merc.s.; Rhus t.*

Selfish – *Sulph.*
Sensitive – *Phos.; Sil.*
  Over – *Nux v.*
Sinking feeling, mid-morning – *Sulph.*
Spiteful – *Nux v.*
Sullen – *Nux v.*
Suspicious – *Lach.*
Sympathetic – *Caust.*
Sympathy, loves – *Puls.*
Sympathy, worse for – *Sep.*

Tearful – *Puls.*

43

Temperament mild – *Puls.*
Tension – *Acon.*
Time passes slowly – *Arg.n.*
Timid – *Caust.*

Untidy – *Sulph.*

Weakness – *Amm.c.; Lyc.; Merc.s.; Nat.m.;*
  Phos.; Sep.
Weariness – *Nat.m.; Sep.*
Weeps when hearing music – *Graph.*
Weeps when telling symptoms – *Sep.*
Weeps when thanked – *Lyc.*
Worry – *Ars.a.*

Yielding – *Sil.*

CHARACTERISTICS –
GENERAL

Acuteness of senses – *Bell.*
Alcohol intolerance – *Sil.*
Anaemia – *Amm.c.*
Assimilation imperfect – *Sil.*
Averse to washing – *Sulph.*

Ball sensation in inner parts – *Sep.*
Bites teeth – *Phyt.*
Bloated after little food – *Lyc.*
Body, lower part dropsical; upper part thin
  – *Lyc.*
Breathless – *Calc.c.*

Chilly when very ill – *Nux v.*
Cold drinks vomited – *Phos.*
Cold but craves air – *Graph.; Sep.*
Costive – *Graph.*
Craves air – *Graph.; Puls.*
Craves eggs – *Calc.c.*
Craves indigestible things – *Calc.c.*
Craves salt – *Nat.m.*
Craves sour things – *Sep.*
Craves sugar – *Arg.n.*
Craves sweets – *Lyc.*
Craves vinegar – *Sep.*

Discharge acrid – *Sulph.*
Discharge burning – *Ars.a.*
Discharge excoriating – *Sulph.*
Discharge jelly-like – *Kali c.*

Discharge offensive – *Sulph.*
Discharge stringy – *Kali b.*
Discharge tough – *Kali b.*
Distension – *Lyc.*
Dizziness – *Gels.*
Drowsiness – *Gels.*

Eruptions oozing sticky substance – *Graph.*
Exhaustion – *Ars.a.*

Faintness kneeling – *Sep.*
Fat – *Calc.c.; Graph.*
Flabby – *Amm.c.; Calc.c.*
Flatulence – *Lyc.*
Fullness, feeling of – *Lyc.*

Grit, lacks physical – *Sil.*

Haemorrhages – *Phos.*
Hunger, gnawing – *Sep.*

Light, intolerance of – *Graph.*
Limbs, heavy – *Gels.*
Loquacity – *Lach.*

Mouth offensive – *Merc.s.*
Mouthsful few, feels full – *Lyc.*
Mucous membranes dry – *Nat.m.*

Nosebleed while washing face – *Amm.c.*

Obesity – *Graph.*
Onset sudden – *Bell.*
Onset violent – *Bell.*
Orifices red – *Sulph.*

Pains burning – *Ars.a.; Bell.; Caust.; Phos.*
Pain burning, worse heat – *Ars.a.*
Pains cutting – *Kali c.*
Pains sharp – *Kali c.*
Pains sore – *Caust.*
Pains small spots, in – *Kali b.*
Pains splinter-like – *Nit.a.*
Pains stitching – *Kali c.*
Pains throbbing – *Bell.*

Pains in occiput over to right eye – *Sang.*
Pains right arm – *Sang.*
Pains right shoulder – *Sang.*
Pains travel upwards – *Sep.*
Paralysis, motor – *Gels.*
Paralysis of single parts – *Caust.*
Prostration – *Ars.a.*
Prostration muscular – *Gels.*
Pupils dilated – *Bell.*

Quick in movement – *Nux v.*

Redness – *Bell.*
Rubbed, desires to be – *Phos.*

Salivation with intense thirst – *Merc.s.*
Sinking feeling mid-morning – *Sulph.*
Skin burning – *Bell.; Sulph.*
Skin cracks – *Graph.*
Skin dry – *Bell.*
Skin eruptions worse winter – *Petr.*
Skin hot – *Bell.*
Skin itching – *Sulph.*
Skin rough – *Graph.*
Sleep, cat-nap – *Sulph.*
Sourness – *Calc.c.*
Sputa offensive – *Sang.*
Stiff on beginning to move – *Rhus t.*
Suppuration – *Sil.*
Sweating, even in cold room – *Calc.c.*
Sweating without relief – *Merc.s.*

Temperature, sudden rise – *Bell.*
Thirst – *Ars.a.; Merc.s.; Nat.m.*
Thirst for cold drinks, vomited as soon as
    warm in stomach – *Phos.*
Thirstless – *Puls.*
Tightness, intolerance of neck – *Lach.*
Tightness, intolerance of waist – *Lach.*
Tiredness – *Gels.*
Tongue, triangular red tip – *Rhus t.*

Trembling – *Gels.; Merc.s.; Phos.*

Washing, dislikes – *Sulph.*
Wind excessive in lower abdomen – *Lyc.*

Yellow saddle across cheeks and nose – *Sep.*

MODALITIES

BETTER

Air, cool – *Puls.*
Air, fresh – *Acon.; Arg.n.; Gels.; Lyc.; Nat.m.*
Applications, hot – *Sep.*

Bathing, cold – *Nat.m.*
Bending forward – *Gels.*

Constipated, when – *Calc.c.*
Covered, being – *Bell.*

Dark, in the – *Calc.c.; Graph.*
Discharge, appearance of – *Lach.*

Erect, being semi – *Bell.*
Eructations, from – *Arg.n.*
Exercise – *Sep.*

Head, wrapping up – *Sil.*
Limbs, drawing up – *Calc.c.*
Loosening garments – *Calc.c.*
Lying on back – *Calc.c.*
Lying on painful side – *Amm.c.*

Motion – *Gels.; Kali c.; Lyc.; Rhus t.*

Nap, after – *Nux v.*

Pressure – *Arg.n.; Sep.*

Rubbing, from – *Calc.c.*

Sweating – *Nat.m.*

Time, breakfast, after – *Calc.c.*

Time, evening – *Nux v.*

Urination, profuse (headache) – *Gels.*

Walking in fresh air – *Puls.*
Warm applications – *Lach.*
Warm drink – *Lyc.*
Warm food – *Lyc.*
Warmth – *Ars.a.; Caust.; Rhus t.; Sil.*
Warmth of bed – *Sep.*
Wrapping up – *Graph.*

MODALITIES

WORSE

Bathing – *Calc.c.*

Clothes, pressure of – *Calc.c.*
Cold applications – *Amm.c.; Ars.a.*
Cold drinks – *Ars.a.; Lyc.*
Cold food – *Arg.n.; Lyc.*
Consolation – *Nat.m.*
Constriction – *Lach.*

Drinking, over – *Nux v.*

Eating, after – *Arg.n.*
Eating, over – *Nux v.*
Exertion, mental – *Calc.c.; Phos.*
Exertion, physical – *Calc.c.; Phos.*
Excitement – *Gels.*

Food, fat – *Puls.*
Food, rich – *Puls.*
Food, sweets – *Arg.n.*

Jar – *Bell.*

Limbs hanging down – *Calc.c.*
Lying down – *Bell.; Rhus t.*
Lying on left side – *Kali c.*
Lying on painful side – *Phos.*
Lying on right side – *Merc.s.*

Menstrual period – *Arg.n.*
Moon, new – *Calc.c.*
Motion – *Phyt.*

51

Move, beginning to – *Rhus t.*
Music – *Nat.m.*

News, bad – *Gels.*
Noise – *Bell.; Nat.m.*

Oysters – *Lyc.*

Sea-shore – *Nat.m.*
Sides of body, left – *Arg.n.; Lach.; Sep.*
Sides of body, right – *Lyc.; Sang.*
Sitting – *Rhus t.*
Sleep – *Lach.*
Standing – *Sulph.*
Stooping – *Calc.c.*
Sweating – *Merc.s.; Rhus t.*
Sweating, after – *Sep.*

Time, morning – *Calc.c.; Kali b.; Nux v.; Sil.; Sulph.*
Time, 10 a.m. – *Gels.*
Time, 10 a.m. – 11 a.m. – *Nat.m.*
Time, after 3 p.m. – *Bell.*
Time, 4 p.m. – 8 p.m. – *Lyc.*
Time, evening – *Amm.c.; Phos.*
Time, midnight – *Acon.*
Time, midnight, after – *Bell.; Calc.c.*
Time, night – *Arg.n.; Ars.a.; Graph.; Merc.s.*
Time, 3 a.m. – *Kali c.*
Time, 3 a.m. – 4 a.m. – *Amm.c.*
Time, waking, on – *Calc.c.; Lach.*
Touch – *Bell.*
Touched, hates to be – *Kali c.*
Trembling – *Phos.*
Twilight – *Phos.*

Uncovering – *Bell.; Sil.*
Undressing – *Kali b.*

Warm drinks – *Phos.*
Warm food – *Phos.*
Warm room – *Acon.; Lyc.; Puls.*

Warmth – *Arg.n.; Graph.; Puls.*
Warmth of bed – *Merc.s.; Sulph.*
Water, working in – *Calc.c.*

MODALITIES – WEATHER

WORSE

Change of weather – *Phos.*
Cold – *Acon.; Ars.a.; Calc.c.; Caust.; Kali c.;
Nit.a.; Nux v.; Sep.*
Cold wet – *Amm.c.; Calc.c.; Rhus t.*
Cold dry winds – *Caust.; Nux v.*
Cold winds – *Acon.; Sep.*

Damp – *Gels.; Sep.; Sil.*

Hot weather – *Graph.; Kali b.; Nit.a.; Puls.*

Spring – *Lach.*
Sultry, moist – *Sep.*

Wet – *Ars.a.*
Wet, getting – *Rhus t.*
Winter – *Petr.*

BETTER

Cold weather – *Arg.n.*

Damp, wet – *Caust.*
Dry – *Amm.c.; Rhus t.*
Dry, warm – *Calc.c.; Sulph.*

Heat – *Kali b.; Phos.*
Humid weather – *Sil.*

Summer – *Petr.; sil.*

Warm, moist – *Kali c.*
Warm, wet – *Nux v.*
Wet – *Sil.*

EARS

SYMPTOMS

Boils: *Merc.s.*

Discharge: –
  Bland: *Puls.*
  Bloody: *Merc.s.; Rhus t.*
  Fetid: *Kali b.; Sil.*
  Offensive: *Lyc.; Merc.s.; Puls.*
  Purulent: *Ars.a.; Calc.c.; Lyc.; Puls.; Sulph.*
  Stringy: *Kali b.*
  Tenacious: *Kali b.*
  Thick: *Kali b.; Lyc.; Merc.s.; Puls.*
  Yellow: *Kali b.; Lyc.; Merc.s.*

Dryness: –
  Inner ear: *Graph.*

Eruptions: –
  Behind ears: *Graph.; Petr.; Sep.*
  Behind ears and on: *Calc.c.*
  Eczema: *Petr.*

Glands: –
  Enlarged: *Calc.c.*

Hearing: –
  Impaired: *Ars.a.; Bell.; Calc.c.; Caust.;*
    Graph.; Lyc.; Merc.s.; Nit.a.; Petr.; Phos.;
    Puls.; Sulph.
  Lost: *Arg.n.*

Inflammation: –
  External: *Merc.s.*

Internal: *Bell.; Merc.s.; Puls.; Sulph.*

Itching: *Amm.c.; Kali c.; Nux v.; Petr.*

Noises: –
  Buzzing: *Acon.; Amm.c; Arg.n.; Bell.; Calc.c.; Caust.*
  Cracking in: *Nat.m.; Nit.a.; Petr.*
  Hissing in: *Calc.c.; Graph.*
  Humming in: *Acon.; Bell.; Caust.; Lyc.; Sang.*
  Ringing in: *Acon.; Arg.n.; Ars.a.; Bell.; Calc.c.; Caust.; Kali c.; Nat.m.*
  Roaring in: *Acon.; Ars.a.; Bell.; Calc.c.; Caust.; Kali c.; Lyc.; Nat.m.; Petr.; Sang.; Sil.*
  Sensitive to noise: *Acon.; Nit.a.; Petr.; Sil.*

Pains: –
  Aching: *Acon.; Merc.s.; Puls.; Sang.*
  Boring: *Bell.*
  Burning: *Ars.a.; Caust.; Merc.s.; Sang.*
  Pressing: *Bell.; Caust.; Merc.s.*
  Pulsating: *Calc.c.; Caust.; Merc.s.*
  Shooting: *Phyt.*
  Sore: *Petr.*
  Stinging: *Sulph.*
  Stitching: *Acon.; Arg.n.; Ars.a.; Calc.c.; Caust.; Kali b.; Kali c.*
  Stopped up feeling: *Caust.; Lyc.; Merc.s.; Puls.; Rhus t.*
  Swallowing, on: *Gels.*
  Tearing: *Acon.; Arg.n.; Ars.a.; Bell.; Caust.; Kali b.; Lach.; Lyc.; Merc.s.; Sulph.*
  Throbbing: *Bell.; Calc.c.; Caust.; Sulph.*
  External ear painful: *Acon.*

Polypus: *Calc.c.; Sang.*

Suppuration: *Kali b.*

Swelling: –
  External: *Acon.*
  Internal: *Kali b.*

Wax: –
Accumulation of: *Caust.*
Dry: *Lach.*
Hard: *Lach.*
Offensive: *Caust.*

NOSE

SYMPTOMS

Acne: *Ars.a.*
Coryza: *Acon.; Caust.; Gels.; Kali b.; Lach.; Lyc.*

Discharge: –
Acrid: *Merc.c.; Nux v.; Nit.a.; Phyt.; Sulph.*
Bland: *Puls.; Sep.*
Burning: *Sulph.*
Corrosive: *Merc.s.; Nit.a.*
Crusts (and plugs): *Lyc.; Sil.*
Excoriating: *Ars.a.*
Fetid: *Calc.c.; Merc.s.; Puls.*
Greenish: *Kali b.; Merc.s.; Sep.*
Jelly-like: *Kali b.*
Offensive: *Graph.; Kali b.; Merc.s.; Nit.a.*
Plugs: *Sep.*
Ropy: *Kali b.*
Stringy: *Kali b.*
Thick: *Calc.c.; Kali b.; Kali s.; Puls.*
Tough: *Kali b.*
Water, scalding: *Gels.*
Watery: *Ars.a.; Kali b.; Nat.m.; Nit.a.*
Yellow: *Calc.c.; Kali b.; Kali c.; Merc.c.; Nit.a.; Puls.; Sang.*

Dryness: –
Mucous membranes: *Acon.; Calc.c.; Graph.; Nat.m.*

Epitaxis: *Amm.c.; Ars.a.; Calc.c.; Caust.; Lach.; Merc.s.; Nit.a.; Petr.; Phos.; Rhus t.*

Inflammation: *Kali b.; Sulph.*

Inflammation, frontal sinuses: *Kali b.; Merc.s.*

Itching: *Amm.c.; Arg.n.; Caust.; Sil.*

Mucus: –
Bloody: *Amm.c.; Bell.*
Watery: *Acon.*

Nostrils: –
Burning: *Petr.*
Cracked: *Petr.*
Sore: *Bell.; Calc.c.; Gels.; Graph.; Kali c.; Merc.s.; Puls.; Sep.*

Pain: –
Nasal bones: *Merc.s.*
Nose, root of: *Acon.; Kali b.; Puls.; Sep.*
Pressing: *Puls.*

Polypi: *Calc.c.; Phos.; Sang.; Sulph.*

Sensation: –
Burning: *Acon.; Ars.a.*
Splinter-like: *Nit.a.*
Tingling: *Acon.*

Septum: –
Perforation: *Sil.*

Smell: –
Acutely sensitive: *Acon.; Graph.; Lyc.; Phos.*
Loss of: *Arg.n.; Kali b.; Puls.; Sil.*

Sneezing: *Acon.; Ars.a.; Calc.c.; Gels.; Kali b.; Lach.; Merc.s.; Nat.m.; Nit.a.; Nux v., Rhus t.; Sil.; Sulph.*

Snuffles: *Amm.c.; Kali b.; Nux v.*

Stopped up: *Acon.; Amm.c.; Ars.a.; Calc.c.; Caust.; Gels.; Graph.; Kali b.; Kali c.; Lyc.; Nat.m.; Nux v.; Rhus t.; Sil.; Sulph.*

Swollen: – *Bell.; Kali c.; Lyc.; Merc.s.; Sep.; Sulph.*

Swollen: – root: *Calc.c.*

Ulcerated: *Calc.c.; Kali c.; Lyc.; Merc.s.; Nit.a.; Petr.; Sep.*

Ulcerated: *Calc.c.; Kali c.; Lyc.; Merc.s.; Nit.a.; Petr.; Sep.*

Ulcerated Septum: *Kali b.*

THROAT

SYMPTOMS

Aphonia: –
  Catarrhal: *Gels.*
  Nervous: *Gels.*

Diphtheria: *Lyc.; Phyt.*

Goitre: *Calc.c.*

Hawking: *Arg. n.; Calc.c.; Nat.m.; Nit.a.*

Hoarseness: *Acon.; Amm.c.; Caust.; Graph.;*
Kali b.; Nat.m.

Inflammation: *Acon.; Bell.; Gels.; Kali b.;*
Nit.a.; Rhus t.; Phyt.; Sulph.

Itching: –
  Soft palate: *Gels.*

Larynx: –
  Sensitive: *Acon.*
  Sore: *Caust.*

Mucus: –
  Gelatinous: *Kali b.*
  Stringy: Kali b.
  Tenacious: *Arg.n.*
  Thick: *Arg.n.; Kali b.*
  Tough: *Kali b.*

Mumps: *Phyt.*

Pain: –
  Burning: *Acon.; Amm.c.; Ars.a.; Caust.;*
    Merc.c.; Phyt.; Sang.; Sulph.
  Pricking: *Sil.*
  Shooting: *Phyt.*
  Smarting: *Acon.; Merc.s.; Phyt.*
  Sore: *Amm.c.; Arg.n.; Bell.; Caust.; Gels.;*
    Lach.; Merc.s.; Nux v.; Phyt.; Puls.; Rhus t.
  Sticking: *Rhus t.*
  Stinging: *Kali c.; Nit.a.; Sil.*
  Stitching: *Calc.c.; Lyc.; Merc.s.*
  Tingling: *Acon.*
  Root of tongue: *Phyt.*

Pharyngitis: *Phyt.*

Parotitis: *Rhus t.*

Quinsy: *Lach.; Merc.s.; Phyt.; Sil.*

Sensations: –
  Dryness: *Acon.; Bell.; Caust.; Kali b.; Kali c.;*
    Lach.; Lyc.; Merc.s.; Nit.a.; Phyt.; Puls.;
    Rhus t.; Sang.; Sulph.
  Constriction: *Acon.; Bell.; Nux v.; Sang.*
  Of lump: *Gels.; Nat.m.; Phyt.; Sulph.*
  Raw: *Amm.c.; Arg.n.; Bell.; Caust.; Lach.;*
    Merc.s.; Nux v.; Puls.
  Rough: *Caust.; Kali b.; Kali c.; Nux v.; Phyt.*
  Scraped: *Nux v.*
  Splinter, of: *Arg.n.; Kali c.; Nit.a.; Sulph.*

Swollen: –
  Cervical glands: *Sil.*
  Parotid glands: *Kali b.; Sil.*
  Sub-maxillary glands: *Calc.c.*
  Palate:*Sulph.*
  Uvula: *Calc.c.*
  Glands: *Ars.a.; Lach.; Merc.s.; Nit.a.; Nux v.;*
    Rhus t.; Sang.

Swallowing: –
  Difficult: *Ars.a.; Bell.; Calc.c.; Gels.; Kali c.; Nit.a.; Phyt.*
  Inclination to: *Bell.*
  Spasm trying to: *Bell.*

Tonsils: –
  Dry: *Acon.*
  Enlarged: *Amm.c.; Bell.*
  Suppuration of: *Lyc.; Merc.s.*
  Swollen: *Acon.; Calc.c.; Lyc.; Nit.a.; Phyt.; Sulph.*
  Ulcerated: *Amm.c.; Nit.a.*

Ulceration: *Lach.; Merc.s.; Phyt.; Sang.*
  Deep ulcers in fauces; *Kali b.*
  Small ulcers: *Calc.c.*
  Of vocal bands: *Lyc.*

Voice:
  Loss of: *Merc.s.; Phyt.*

A FEW NOTES
ABOUT FOOD

Our daily food is very important and it seems appropriate to have a look at what we eat in view of all the reports in the daily press about food poisoning, contamination and so on.

'Anything for quickness' seems to be the rule of so many housewives who have a family to cater for and maybe a job as well, either part or full time.

But good health is not supported by tinned and packaged foods, take-aways and fry-ups! I am sure that micro-wave ovens are not good although they are incredibly quick. A doctor in America reports that 2000 cases of cataract have been traced to the constant use of micro-wave ovens and a report in the 'Daily Telegraph' on the 11th July 1989 was headed '97% ignorant of food poison risks from micro-waves'. I feel sure that we shall hear more adverse reports in the future.

Our food should be as fresh as possible and 'whole'. Bread made from 100% wholemeal flour contains the germ of the wheat and roughage − it is delicious.

The ingredients on all packets of cereals should be read carefully and only those without sugar and/or added vitamins selected. We all need vitamins but they should be chosen for the individual, if there is a shortage, and they should always be made from natural sources. Porridge made from oatmeal and sweetened with a little honey is very good and a health giving breakfast.

Sugar should be taken in strict moderation and only Barbados used. Far too much white sugar is consumed; it has a very acid reaction which can cause trouble. These remarks apply especially to children who often consume fruit drinks with added sugar, lots of sweets and ice creams. These should be cut to the minimum. Fresh or dried fruits are a very good substitute.

Honey is better than sugar although this should be taken with discretion; honey is a natural substance but, nevertheless, it is still sugar.

And whilst we are talking about sugar it is unwise to switch to artificial sweeteners for drinks.

Where possible it is better to obtain organically grown vegetables, salads and fruit although this can be difficult as most are sprayed and grown in soil to which fertilisers have been added.

A vegetarian diet is recommended but if meat is enjoyed lamb, or poultry from free-range chickens or fish are better than red-meat.

Vegetarians have a good variety of cheese, especially cottage, nuts, whole rice and wholemeal pasta for dishes which can be taken with cooked vegetables or salad. It is advisable to eat as much raw food as possible because cooking, even steaming, destroys some of the vitamins through the high temperature.

Aluminium saucepans should be avoided and replaced by stainless steel or enamel. We have heard a great deal about aluminium poisoning recently following the Camelford disaster; homoeopaths have been able to deal successfully with the effects of aluminium poisoning for very many years!

All dairy foods should be taken in moderation and milk reduced to minimum requirements.

Herbal teas are a good substitute for tea and coffee, and drinks made from Vecon or Marmite are delicious, especially in cold weather.

The above hints point in the direction of fitness but special diets may be needed in some illnesses and many books are available on food and diets.

However, for acute conditions, especially of the ear, nose and throat when catarrhal problems often occur, all dairy produce should be avoided and a cleansing diet taken for a few days, consisting mostly of fruit and salads.

If acute conditions commence with a fever (or, of course, if a fever develops) no food should be taken until it has subsided, but drinking plenty of fluids is essential. This applies especially to children. So many mothers have told me that they have done everything to make their child eat at such a time; they are so much better without food and will usually ask for something when the fever has abated. I mention this because in my experience many people are terrified that they will become weak and faint if they go without food for a day.

It is hard work these days to procure nourishing food but I can promise that the effort is worthwhile, and remember, homoeopathic remedies cannot compensate for junk food.

GLOSSARY OF
MEDICAL TERMS

Alae nasi	The outer side of external nostrils
Cervical	Pertaining to the neck
Coryza	Nasal catarrh (cold in the head)
Epitaxis	Bleeding from the nose
Eustachian tube	The canal from throat to ear
Fauces	The short passage between the back of the mouth and the pharynx
Meatus	An opening into a passage
Meniere's Disease	Giddiness resulting from disease of the internal ear or the equilibrating mechanism of the brain
Nares	Nostrils
Occiput	Back of head
Otitis media	Inflammation of middle ear
Otorrhoea	A purulent discharge from the ear
Parotid	Salivary gland under the ear
Rhinitis	Inflammation of the nose

Submaxillary	Under the lower jaw
Tinnitus airium	Ringing in the ears